Renal Diet cookbook for seniors

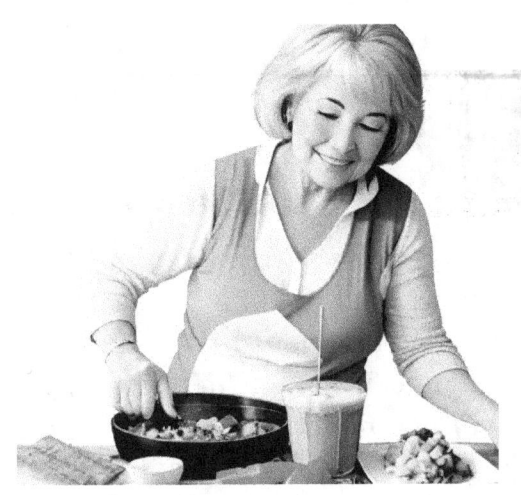

The complete comprehensive guide to managing incurable kidney disease with easy and tasty recipes low in sodium, potassium, phosphorus and 30-day meal plans

Dr. Stephen Campbell

Table of contents

Introduction

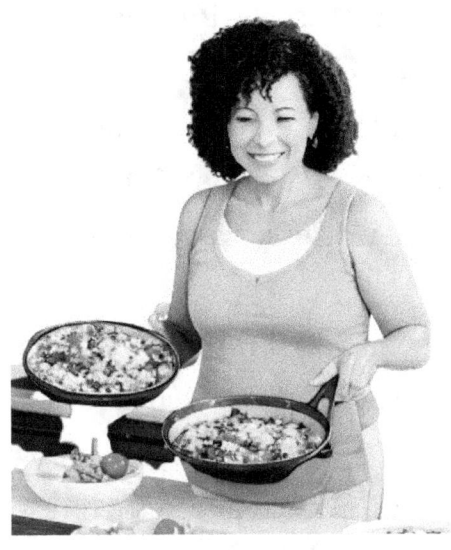

The "Renal Diet Cookbook for Seniors" is a comprehensive guide that offers a wide array of delicious and nourishing recipes specifically designed for individuals with renal issues. As we age, our kidneys undergo changes, and maintaining kidney health becomes crucial for overall well-being. This cookbook aims to provide seniors with practical, easy-to-follow recipes that promote kidney health while still satisfying the taste buds.

Meet Eleanor. She was a 75-year-old woman who had been diagnosed with stage 2 kidney disease. She was taking medication to control her condition, but she knew that she needed to make some changes to her diet if she wanted to prevent her kidney disease from progressing.

One day, Eleanor was browsing through the library when she came across a cookbook called "The Renal Diet" She was intrigued by the book, so she checked it out and started reading.

The book was full of delicious recipes that were specifically designed for people with kidney disease. Eleanor was amazed at how many different and flavorful dishes she could make that were also good for her kidneys.

She started following the recipes in the book, and within a few weeks, she started to feel better. Her energy levels increased, and she had less fatigue. Her blood work also showed that her kidney function was improving.

Eleanor was so grateful for the cookbook that she decided to share it with other people who were struggling with kidney disease. She started a blog and a website where she shared her story and the recipes from the cookbook.

Her blog and website quickly became popular, and she started receiving emails from people all over the world who were thanking her for helping them to improve their health.

Eleanor was so happy that she had found the cookbook that had saved her life. She knew that she was making a difference in the lives of others, and she was determined to continue her work to help people with kidney disease live healthier lives.

Chapter 1: Understanding Renal Diets

1.1 What is a Renal Diet?

A renal diet, also known as a kidney diet, is a specialized eating plan designed to promote kidney health and manage the progression of kidney disease. It focuses on controlling the intake of certain nutrients, such as sodium, potassium, phosphorus, and protein, which can negatively impact kidney function when consumed in excessive amounts. By following a renal diet, individuals can support their kidneys' ability to filter waste products and maintain electrolyte balance.

1.2 Goals of a Renal Diet

The primary goals of a renal diet are to:

Manage fluid balance: Kidneys play a crucial role in regulating fluid levels in the body. A renal diet aims to control fluid intake, preventing fluid overload and maintaining optimal hydration.

Control blood pressure: High blood pressure is a common complication of kidney disease. A renal diet emphasizes reducing sodium intake, as excessive sodium can lead to fluid retention and increased blood pressure.

Limit sodium intake: Sodium is an essential mineral, but excessive consumption can strain the kidneys. A renal diet provides strategies for reducing sodium intake and highlights alternative ways to enhance flavor without relying on salt.

Regulate potassium levels: Potassium is a mineral that, in excess, can be harmful to individuals with kidney issues. A renal diet provides guidance on managing potassium intake, ensuring it remains within a safe range.

Monitor phosphorus intake: The kidneys help regulate phosphorus levels in the body. When kidneys are compromised, excess phosphorus can accumulate, leading to bone and heart problems. A renal diet educates individuals about phosphorus-rich foods and suggests alternatives to control phosphorus intake.

Optimize protein intake: Protein is necessary for overall health, but excessive protein consumption can burden the kidneys. A renal diet recommends appropriate protein amounts and offers sources that are easier for the kidneys to process.

1.3 Food Groups in a Renal Diet

Chapter 1 explores the various food groups that are part of a renal diet, including:

High-quality protein sources: Discover lean sources of protein that are gentle on the kidneys, such as fish, poultry, eggs, and tofu. We provide delicious recipes that incorporate these protein sources while considering their impact on renal health.

Low-sodium alternatives: Learn about flavorful herbs, spices, and salt substitutes that can be used in place of traditional high-sodium seasonings. We share tips on reading food labels and making informed choices to reduce sodium content in your meals.

Kidney-friendly fruits and vegetables: Explore a wide range of fruits and vegetables that are low in potassium and phosphorus but rich in essential vitamins and minerals. We offer creative ways to incorporate these nutrient-packed ingredients into your diet.

Whole grains and carbohydrates: Discover the importance of choosing whole grains and low-glycemic index carbohydrates for sustained energy and overall health. We provide a list of renal-friendly grains and carbohydrate options to diversify your meals.

Fluid management: Learn techniques to effectively manage fluid intake, including monitoring fluid balance, choosing appropriate beverages, and managing thirst. We offer practical tips to help you maintain optimal hydration without straining your kidneys.

Chapter 2: Essential Nutrients for Kidney Health

2.1 Protein: The Building Block of Kidney Health

Protein is an essential nutrient that supports the growth, repair, and maintenance of body tissues, including the kidneys. However, for individuals with kidney issues, it's important to consume the right amount of protein to minimize stress on the kidneys. In this chapter, we discuss the concept of high-quality protein and provide a list of kidney-friendly protein sources. You'll find recipes that showcase these protein-rich ingredients while maintaining a balanced renal diet.

2.2 Sodium: Balancing Fluids and Blood Pressure

Sodium, commonly found in table salt and processed foods, can contribute to fluid retention and high blood pressure, both of which can negatively impact kidney function. Discover the importance of reducing sodium intake in a renal diet and learn practical strategies for flavoring your meals without relying on excessive salt. We'll guide you through the process of reading food labels and identifying hidden sources of sodium, ensuring that you make informed choices to support your kidney health.

2.3 Potassium: Managing Electrolyte Balance

An electrolyte that helps control fluid balance, neuron activity, and muscle contractions is potassium. However, individuals with kidney issues may experience difficulty in balancing potassium levels. In this chapter, we provide a comprehensive list of low-potassium foods, as well as tips for controlling potassium intake. You'll explore delicious recipes that incorporate these low-potassium ingredients, ensuring a healthy and well-balanced diet.

2.4 Phosphorus: Maintaining Bone Health

Phosphorus is another essential mineral that plays a crucial role in bone health. However, excessive phosphorus levels can lead to complications for individuals with kidney problems. Learn about phosphorus-rich foods and their impact on kidney health. We provide alternatives and strategies for managing phosphorus intake while still enjoying tasty and nutritious meals.

2.5 Fluid Intake: Balancing Hydration

Managing fluid intake is an important aspect of kidney health, as excessive fluid consumption can strain the kidneys. In this chapter, we discuss the importance of monitoring fluid balance and offer practical tips for managing thirst without compromising hydration. You'll find refreshing beverage recipes and ideas to keep your fluid intake in check while enjoying flavorful and satisfying drinks.

2.6 Micronutrients: Supporting Overall Health

Beyond the essential macronutrients, a renal diet should also address the importance of micronutrients. We explore key vitamins and minerals that support overall health and kidney function. From vitamin B12 to iron, we provide insights into their roles and suggest food sources that are compatible with a renal diet. Ensuring that your meals are nutritionally balanced will contribute to your overall well-being.

Chapter 3: Renal-Friendly Breakfast Recipes

3.1 Vegetable Egg White Omelet

Kickstart your morning with a protein-packed vegetable egg white omelet. This recipe combines fluffy egg whites with a colorful medley of kidney-friendly vegetables, such as bell peppers, spinach, and mushrooms. Seasoned with herbs and spices, this omelet is a delightful and satisfying way to begin your day.

3.2 Creamy Oatmeal with Berries

Indulge in a warm and comforting bowl of creamy oatmeal topped with a generous handful of antioxidant-rich berries. This recipe utilizes low-fat milk or a dairy alternative, along with a touch of sweetness from a natural sugar substitute. It's a hearty and filling breakfast option that will keep you satisfied throughout the morning.

3.3 Whole Grain Pancakes with Applesauce

Enjoy a stack of fluffy whole grain pancakes that are both kidney-friendly and delicious. These pancakes are made with a combination of whole wheat flour and oat flour, providing fiber and nutrients. Instead of traditional syrup, top them with unsweetened applesauce for a naturally sweet and flavorful twist.

3.4 Yogurt Parfait with Nuts and Seeds

Create a refreshing and protein-rich yogurt parfait by layering low-fat yogurt with a variety of kidney-friendly nuts and seeds. Walnuts, almonds, chia seeds, and flaxseeds provide a satisfying crunch while adding healthy fats and essential nutrients. Top it off with a sprinkle of cinnamon for an extra burst of flavor.

3.5 Spinach and Mushroom Breakfast Wrap

Wrap up a nutritious breakfast with this spinach and mushroom breakfast wrap. Sautéed spinach, mushrooms, and onions are combined with scrambled eggs and wrapped in a whole wheat tortilla. This portable and filling meal is perfect for those busy mornings when you're on the go.

3.6 Fruit Smoothie Bowl

Indulge in a refreshing and vibrant fruit smoothie bowl packed with kidney-friendly fruits like berries, bananas, and melons. Blend the fruits with a splash of low-fat milk or a dairy alternative until smooth, and then top it with a variety of renal-friendly toppings such as chopped nuts, unsweetened coconut flakes, and a drizzle of honey.

3.7 Quinoa Breakfast Bowl

Start your day with a nutritious and protein-rich quinoa breakfast bowl. Cooked quinoa is combined with kidney-friendly fruits, such as diced apples, berries, and a sprinkle of cinnamon. Add a dollop of low-fat yogurt or a dairy alternative for creaminess and top it off with a sprinkle of toasted almonds for a delightful crunch.

3.8 Sweet Potato Hash with Poached Eggs

Experience a savory and satisfying breakfast with this sweet potato hash topped with perfectly poached eggs. The sweet potatoes are seasoned with herbs and spices, then sautéed until tender and golden. The dish is completed with a perfectly poached egg on top, creating a protein-rich and flavorful morning meal

Chapter 4: Nourishing Lunch Ideas

4.1 Grilled Chicken Salad with Citrus Dressing

Enjoy a refreshing and protein-packed grilled chicken salad with a tangy citrus dressing. Grilled chicken breast is paired with a colorful mix of kidney-friendly vegetables, such as cucumbers, cherry tomatoes, and bell peppers. Tossed in a light and zesty citrus dressing, this salad is a flavorful and nutritious lunch option.

4.2 Lentil Soup with Vegetables

Savor a hearty and fiber-rich lentil soup loaded with kidney-friendly vegetables. This comforting soup combines nutritious lentils with a medley of vegetables like carrots, celery, and onions. Seasoned with herbs and spices, it's a satisfying and nourishing option for a well-rounded lunch.

4.3 Quinoa and Vegetable Stir-Fry

Whip up a quick and nutritious quinoa and vegetable stir-fry that is packed with flavors and essential nutrients. This recipe combines protein-rich quinoa with an array of kidney-friendly vegetables, such as broccoli, bell peppers, and snap peas. Seasoned with a flavorful sauce, this stir-fry will leave you feeling satisfied and energized.

4.4 Tuna and White Bean Salad

Indulge in a protein-rich tuna and white bean salad that is both satisfying and kidney-friendly. This recipe combines flaked tuna with white beans, cherry tomatoes, red onions, and fresh herbs. Tossed in a light lemon vinaigrette, it's a refreshing and filling option for a healthy lunch.

4.5 Baked Salmon with Roasted Vegetables

Treat yourself to a succulent baked salmon fillet paired with a colorful assortment of roasted vegetables. The salmon is seasoned with herbs and spices and baked to perfection, while the roasted vegetables, such as asparagus, zucchini, and cherry tomatoes, add a burst of flavor and nutrients to the dish.

4.6 Vegetable and Bean Wrap

Wrap up a nutritious and fiber-rich lunch with a vegetable and bean wrap. Load a whole wheat tortilla with kidney-friendly vegetables like lettuce, cucumbers, tomatoes, and a mix of kidney beans and black beans. Add a dollop of low-fat yogurt or a kidney-friendly dressing for extra creaminess and flavor.

4.7 Quinoa Stuffed Bell Peppers

Experience a satisfying and nutrient-dense lunch with quinoa-stuffed bell peppers. Roasted bell peppers are filled with a flavorful mixture of quinoa, kidney-friendly vegetables, and herbs. Baked to perfection, these stuffed peppers make for a visually appealing and delicious meal.

4.8 Turkey and Avocado Lettuce Wraps

Indulge in a light and refreshing lunch with turkey and avocado lettuce wraps. Use large lettuce leaves as a wrap and fill them with lean turkey slices, avocado, and kidney-friendly vegetables. Drizzle with a tangy dressing or mustard for added flavor.

Chapter 5: Wholesome Dinner Recipes

5.1 Baked Herb Chicken with Roasted Vegetables

Indulge in a flavorful and tender baked herb chicken served with a side of colorful roasted vegetables. The chicken is marinated with herbs and spices, then baked to perfection, while the roasted vegetables, such as carrots, broccoli, and cauliflower, add a delicious touch of sweetness and texture to the dish.

5.2 Shrimp and Vegetable Stir-Fry

Savor a protein-packed shrimp and vegetable stir-fry that bursts with flavors. This recipe combines succulent shrimp with a variety of kidney-friendly vegetables like bell peppers, snap peas, and mushrooms. Stir-fried in a savory sauce, it's a quick and nutritious dinner option that will leave you feeling satisfied.

5.3 Quinoa-Stuffed Zucchini Boats

Experience a creative and nutritious dinner with quinoa-stuffed zucchini boats. Halved zucchini are hollowed out and filled with a flavorful mixture of cooked quinoa, kidney beans, diced tomatoes, and herbs. Baked to perfection, these zucchini boats are both visually appealing and packed with essential nutrients.

5.4 Baked Cod with Herbed Quinoa Pilaf

Enjoy a delicate and flaky baked cod filet served with a side of herbed quinoa pilaf. The cod is seasoned with herbs and lemon juice, then baked to perfection. The quinoa pilaf is cooked with kidney-friendly vegetables, such as bell peppers and onions, and flavored with aromatic herbs for a delightful and well-rounded meal.

5.5 Turkey Meatballs with Tomato Sauce and Whole Wheat Pasta

Delight in a comforting plate of turkey meatballs smothered in a flavorful tomato sauce, served over whole wheat pasta. These turkey meatballs are made with lean ground turkey, kidney-friendly breadcrumbs, and a blend of herbs and spices. Paired with a whole wheat pasta of your choice, it's a satisfying and kidney-friendly dinner option.

5.6 Vegetable Curry with Brown Rice

Experience the aromatic flavors of a vegetable curry served with fluffy brown rice. This kidney-friendly curry is made with a medley of vegetables like carrots, bell peppers, cauliflower, and kidney beans, simmered in a fragrant blend of spices and coconut milk. Serve it over brown rice for a wholesome and satisfying dinner.

5.7 Beef Stir-Fry with Broccoli and Snow Peas

Indulge in a savory beef stir-fry loaded with kidney-friendly vegetables. Sliced beef is stir-fried with broccoli, snow peas, and onions in a flavorful sauce, creating a protein-rich and nutrient-dense dinner option. Pair it with brown rice or quinoa for a complete meal.

5.8 Lentil and Vegetable Curry

Savor a hearty and aromatic lentil and vegetable curry that is both satisfying and kidney-friendly. This curry features lentils, kidney-friendly vegetables, and a blend of spices simmered in a tomato-based sauce. Serve it over brown rice or with whole wheat bread for a delicious and nourishing dinner.

Chapter 6: Satisfying Snacks and Appetizers

6.1 Roasted Chickpeas

Enjoy a crunchy and protein-packed snack with roasted chickpeas. Simply toss canned chickpeas with a drizzle of olive oil and your choice of kidney-friendly seasonings, such as cumin, paprika, or garlic powder. Roast them in the oven until crispy, and you'll have a flavorful and nutritious snack to munch on.

6.2 Greek Yogurt Dip with Fresh Vegetables

Dip into a creamy and tangy Greek yogurt dip accompanied by a colorful assortment of fresh vegetables. Mix low-fat Greek yogurt with herbs and spices like dill, garlic, and lemon juice for a refreshing and protein-rich dip. Serve it alongside sliced cucumbers, bell peppers, cherry tomatoes, and celery sticks for a wholesome and kidney-friendly snack.

6.3 Baked Tortilla Chips with Salsa

Satisfy your craving for chips and dip with homemade baked tortilla chips and a kidney-friendly salsa. Cut whole wheat tortillas into triangles, lightly coat them with olive oil, and bake until crispy. Pair them with a salsa made from diced tomatoes, onions, cilantro, lime juice, and kidney-friendly seasonings. It's a guilt-free snack option that's full of flavor.

6.4 Cottage Cheese and Fruit Parfait

Indulge in a creamy and fruity cottage cheese parfait that provides a combination of protein and natural sweetness. Layer low-fat cottage cheese with kidney-friendly fruits like berries, diced peaches, or melon in a glass. Sprinkle some chopped nuts or a drizzle of honey on top for added texture and flavor.

6.5 Veggie Sticks with Hummus

Crunch on a colorful medley of veggie sticks paired with a creamy and protein-rich hummus. Slice kidney-friendly vegetables like carrots, celery, bell peppers, and cucumbers into sticks. Dip them into a homemade or store-bought kidney-friendly hummus for a satisfying and nutritious snack.

6.6 Smoked Salmon Cucumber Bites

Experience a burst of flavors with smoked salmon cucumber bites. Slice cucumbers into rounds and top each one with a small piece of smoked salmon, a dollop of low-fat cream cheese, and a sprinkle of fresh dill. These bite-sized delights are not only refreshing but also packed with essential nutrients.

6.7 Edamame Salad

Enjoy a protein-rich and refreshing edamame salad as a light and nutritious snack. Toss cooked and shelled edamame beans with kidney-friendly vegetables like cherry tomatoes, cucumber, red onion, and a light vinaigrette dressing. It's a vibrant and satisfying snack option that's full of flavor.

6.8 Sweet Potato Fries

Satisfy your craving for fries with a kidney-friendly twist by making sweet potato fries. Slice sweet potatoes into thin strips, toss them with a touch of olive oil and kidney-friendly seasonings like paprika or cinnamon, then bake until crispy. These fries are a healthier alternative that still deliver on taste.

Chapter 7: Flavorful Soups and Salads

7.1 Minestrone Soup

Delight in a hearty and vegetable-packed minestrone soup. This classic Italian soup features kidney-friendly vegetables like carrots, celery, zucchini, and kidney beans, simmered in a flavorful tomato broth. Seasoned with herbs and spices, it's a comforting and nourishing option for a satisfying meal.

7.2 Chicken and Vegetable Soup

Savor a comforting bowl of chicken and vegetable soup that is both filling and kidney-friendly. This recipe combines lean chicken breast with a medley of kidney-friendly vegetables like carrots, celery, and onions. Simmered in a flavorful broth, it's a perfect option for a nourishing and soothing meal.

7.3 Tomato and Cucumber Salad

Indulge in a refreshing and tangy tomato and cucumber salad.Juicy tomatoes, crunchy cucumbers, and finely cut red onions should all be combined. Toss with a light vinaigrette dressing made from kidney-friendly ingredients like lemon juice, olive oil, and herbs. This vibrant salad is a refreshing and hydrating option.

7.4 Lentil and Vegetable Soup

Experience the hearty flavors of a lentil and vegetable soup that is both satisfying and kidney-friendly. This soup combines protein-packed lentils with kidney-friendly vegetables like carrots, celery, and spinach. Infused with aromatic herbs and spices, it's a comforting and nutritious option for a well-rounded meal.

7.5 Greek Salad

Enjoy a classic and refreshing Greek salad bursting with Mediterranean flavors. This salad features crisp lettuce, juicy tomatoes, cucumbers, red onions, and briny olives. Topped with crumbled feta cheese and dressed with a kidney-friendly vinaigrette made from lemon juice, olive oil, and herbs, it's a perfect combination of flavors.

7.6 Butternut Squash Soup

Indulge in the creamy and comforting flavors of butternut squash soup. This velvety soup is made from roasted butternut squash, kidney-friendly spices, and a touch of cream or dairy alternative for richness. It's a delicious and nourishing option for a satisfying meal.

7.7 Spinach Salad with Berries and Almonds

Experience a delightful combination of flavors with a spinach salad topped with kidney-friendly berries and almonds. Combine fresh baby spinach with a mix of kidney-friendly berries like strawberries, blueberries, or raspberries. Sprinkle with toasted almonds and drizzle with a light vinaigrette for a nutritious and vibrant salad.

7.8 Vegetable Barley Soup

Savor the wholesome goodness of a vegetable barley soup packed with kidney-friendly vegetables and fiber-rich barley. This soup combines a variety of vegetables like carrots, peas, and green beans with tender barley, creating a filling and flavorful dish. Seasoned with herbs and spices, it's a nourishing option for a satisfying meal.

Chapter 8: Creative Side Dishes

8.1 Quinoa Pilaf with Roasted Vegetables

Enhance your meal with a colorful and flavorful quinoa pilaf featuring a medley of roasted kidney-friendly vegetables. Roast vegetables like bell peppers, zucchini, and eggplant, then mix them with cooked quinoa and fresh herbs. This side dish is not only visually appealing but also packed with nutrients.

8.2 Mashed Cauliflower

Swap traditional mashed potatoes for a creamy and kidney-friendly alternative—mashed cauliflower. Steam or boil cauliflower florets until tender, then mash them with a touch of low-sodium vegetable broth, herbs, and spices. The result is a satisfying and flavorful side dish that pairs well with a variety of main courses.

8.3 Sautéed Green Beans with Almonds

Elevate simple green beans by sautéing them with sliced almonds and kidney-friendly seasonings. This side dish adds a delightful crunch and nutty flavor to your meal. Sauté the green beans in a small amount of olive oil, then toss them with toasted almonds and a sprinkle of lemon zest for a burst of freshness.

8.4 Roasted Brussels Sprouts with Balsamic Glaze

Discover the irresistible flavors of roasted Brussels sprouts drizzled with a tangy balsamic glaze. Roast Brussels sprouts until they are caramelized and tender, then toss them in a balsamic glaze made from kidney-friendly ingredients like balsamic vinegar, olive oil, and a natural sugar substitute. This side dish is a perfect balance of savory and tangy.

8.5 Herb-Roasted Potatoes

Add a touch of herb-infused deliciousness to your meal with herb-roasted potatoes. Toss small potatoes with kidney-friendly herbs like rosemary, thyme, and garlic, along with a drizzle of olive oil. They should be roasted until the outside is crispy and the inside is tender. These flavorful potatoes are a delightful addition to any main course.

8.6 Steamed Asparagus with Lemon Butter

Enjoy the simplicity of steamed asparagus paired with a tangy and kidney-friendly lemon butter sauce. Steam asparagus until tender-crisp, then drizzle with a sauce made from melted low-sodium butter, freshly squeezed lemon juice, and a sprinkle of lemon zest. This side dish is a perfect combination of vibrant flavors.

8.7 Quinoa and Black Bean Salad

Enhance your meal with a protein-packed quinoa and black bean salad. Mix cooked quinoa with kidney-friendly black beans, diced tomatoes, red onions, and herbs. Dress the salad with a light vinaigrette made from kidney-friendly ingredients like lemon juice, olive oil, and herbs. This side dish adds a satisfying and nutritious element to your plate.

8.8 Grilled Eggplant with Herbs

Elevate your meal with grilled eggplant slices seasoned with kidney-friendly herbs and spices. Brush eggplant slices with a small amount of olive oil, then grill until tender and slightly charred. Sprinkle with herbs like basil, oregano, or thyme, and a squeeze of lemon juice for a burst of freshness. Grilled eggplant is a versatile side dish that pairs well with a variety of main courses.

Chapter 9: Delectable Desserts with Kidney-Friendly Ingredients

9.1 Berry Parfait

Indulge in a refreshing and nutritious berry parfait. Layer kidney-friendly berries like strawberries, blueberries, and raspberries with low-fat yogurt or a dairy alternative. Add a sprinkle of chopped nuts or a drizzle of honey for extra texture and flavor. This parfait is a guilt-free dessert that is packed with antioxidants and natural sweetness.

9.2 Baked Apples with Cinnamon

Experience the warm and comforting flavors of baked apples with a hint of cinnamon. Core apples and fill them with a mixture of kidney-friendly sweeteners like cinnamon, a natural sugar substitute, and a touch of lemon juice. Bake the apples until they are soft and browned. Serve them warm with a dollop of low-fat yogurt or a sprinkle of chopped nuts for a delightful treat.

9.3 Chia Pudding with Fresh Fruit

Delight in a creamy and nutritious chia pudding topped with kidney-friendly fresh fruit. Combine chia seeds with low-fat milk or a dairy alternative, along with a natural sugar substitute and vanilla extract. Allow the mixture to set until it forms a pudding-like consistency. Top it with kidney-friendly fruits like sliced bananas, berries, or diced mango for a delightful and fiber-rich dessert.

9.4 Frozen Banana Bites

Satisfy your sweet cravings with frozen banana bites. Slice bananas into bite-sized pieces and dip them in melted dark chocolate that has been sweetened with a natural sugar substitute. Lay the banana bites on a parchment-lined tray and freeze until the chocolate hardens. These frozen treats offer a creamy and naturally sweet indulgence.

9.5 Yogurt Bark with Nuts and Berries

Create a delightful and protein-rich yogurt bark by spreading low-fat yogurt or a dairy alternative on a baking sheet. Top it with kidney-friendly nuts and berries, such as chopped almonds, walnuts, and blueberries. Freeze until firm, then break it into pieces. This crunchy and creamy dessert is perfect for a refreshing and satisfying treat.

9.6 Lemon Poppy Seed Muffins

Indulge in tangy and moist lemon poppy seed muffins made with kidney-friendly ingredients. These muffins are made with a combination of kidney-friendly flours, natural sugar substitutes, lemon zest, and poppy seeds. They offer a burst of citrus flavor and a delightful texture. Enjoy them as a guilt-free dessert or a sweet snack.

9.7 Frozen Yogurt Bites

Enjoy bite-sized frozen yogurt treats that are both refreshing and kidney-friendly. Drop spoonfuls of low-fat yogurt or a dairy alternative onto a parchment-lined tray and sprinkle with kidney-friendly toppings like chopped fruit or nuts. Freeze until firm, and you'll have a satisfying and cool dessert to enjoy.

9.8 Rice Pudding with Cinnamon

Savor the comforting and creamy flavors of rice pudding seasoned with cinnamon. Use kidney-friendly grains like short-grain white rice or arborio rice, combined with low-fat milk or a dairy alternative, a natural sugar substitute, and a touch of cinnamon. Cook it slowly until the rice is tender and the mixture thickens. Serve it warm or chilled for a delightful and nostalgic dessert.

Chapter 10: Refreshing Kidney-Friendly Beverages

10.1 Infused Water

Stay hydrated with the refreshing flavors of infused water. Simply add kidney-friendly fruits like sliced lemons, limes, cucumbers, or berries to a pitcher of water and let it infuse for a few hours in the refrigerator. This simple yet flavorful beverage will quench your thirst while providing a burst of natural flavor.

10.2 Green Smoothie

Start your day with a nutrient-packed green smoothie that supports kidney health. Blend together kidney-friendly leafy greens like spinach or kale with low-potassium fruits like green apples, kiwi, and cucumbers. Add a splash of water or a dairy alternative, and blend until smooth. This smoothie is loaded with antioxidants, vitamins, and minerals.

10.3 Hibiscus Iced Tea

Sip on a refreshing and kidney-friendly hibiscus iced tea. Steep dried hibiscus petals in hot water until the tea reaches your desired strength, then sweeten with a natural sugar substitute if desired. With a lemon or mint sprig for decoration, pour the tea over ice. Hibiscus tea not only provides a delightful taste but also offers potential health benefits for kidney health.

10.4 Watermelon Lime Cooler

Cool off with a hydrating watermelon lime cooler that is both refreshing and kidney-friendly. Blend fresh watermelon chunks with the juice of lime, a touch of natural sugar substitute, and a few ice cubes. This thirst-quenching beverage offers a natural sweetness and a burst of citrus flavor.

10.5 Iced Herbal Tea

Enjoy a soothing and kidney-friendly iced herbal tea. Brew your favorite kidney-friendly herbal tea, such as mint or chamomile, and let it cool. Pour the tea over ice and sweeten with a natural sugar substitute if desired. This caffeine-free beverage provides a calming and hydrating experience.

10.6 Berry Smoothie

Indulge in a creamy and antioxidant-rich berry smoothie. Blend kidney-friendly berries like strawberries, blueberries, or raspberries with a low-fat yogurt or a dairy alternative, a splash of low-potassium fruit juice, and a natural sugar substitute if desired. This smoothie is a delicious and nutrient-packed treat.

10.7 Cucumber Mint Refresher

Quench your thirst with a revitalizing cucumber mint refresher. Blend cucumber slices with fresh mint leaves, a squeeze of lime juice, and a touch of natural sugar substitute.

Strain the mixture and serve it over ice for a cooling and invigorating beverage.

10.8 Coconut Water Electrolyte Drink

Replenish your electrolytes with a kidney-friendly coconut water drink. Combine natural coconut water with a splash of low-potassium fruit juice and a pinch of sea salt. This hydrating beverage provides essential minerals and a subtle sweetness.

Chapter 11: Lifestyle Tips for Kidney Health

11.1 Stay Hydrated

One of the most important factors in kidney health is maintaining proper hydration. Drink an adequate amount of fluids throughout the day, especially water, to ensure optimal kidney function. Adequate hydration helps flush toxins from the kidneys and promotes overall kidney health. Aim to drink at least 8 cups (64 ounces) of water per day, or as advised by your healthcare provider.

11.2 Regular Exercise

Engaging in regular physical activity is beneficial for kidney health. Exercise improves blood circulation, helps control blood pressure, and reduces the risk of chronic conditions that can impact kidney function, such as diabetes and cardiovascular disease. On most days of the week, try to get in at least 30 minutes of moderate-intensity exercise, such as brisk walking, swimming, or cycling.

11.3 Manage Blood Pressure

Kidney damage has high blood pressure as one of its main causes.Take steps to manage and control your blood pressure within a healthy range. This includes following a balanced diet low in sodium, limiting alcohol consumption, quitting smoking if applicable, and taking prescribed medications as directed by your healthcare provider.

11.4 Avoid Smoking and Limit Alcohol Intake

Alcohol abuse and smoking both have a negative impact on kidney health. Smoking increases the risk of kidney disease and accelerates kidney damage. Alcohol, when consumed in excess, can lead to high blood pressure and liver damage, which can impact kidney function. Quit smoking and limit alcohol intake to promote kidney health.

11.5 Manage Stress Levels

Chronic stress can aggravate kidney problems among other health problems. Find healthy ways to manage and reduce stress in your life, such as practicing relaxation techniques, engaging in hobbies, spending time with loved ones, or seeking support from a mental health professional if needed. Prioritizing stress management can have a positive impact on your overall well-being, including kidney health.

11.6 Regular Health Check-ups

Regular check-ups and screenings are crucial for monitoring your kidney health. Schedule regular visits with your healthcare provider to monitor blood pressure, blood sugar levels, and kidney function. Early detection and intervention can help prevent or manage kidney-related issues effectively.

11.7 Avoid Overuse of Over-the-Counter Medications

Certain over-the-counter medications, such as nonsteroidal anti-inflammatory drugs (NSAIDs), can cause kidney damage when used excessively or for extended periods. Consult with your healthcare provider before taking any new medications, and use over-the-counter medications as directed and only when necessary.

11.8 Maintain a Healthy Weight

Kidney health depends on maintaining a healthy weight. Excess body weight puts strain on the kidneys and can contribute to the development of conditions like diabetes and high blood pressure, which are risk factors for kidney disease. Follow a balanced diet, engage in regular physical activity, and work towards achieving and maintaining a healthy weight range.

Chapter 12: Kidney Health for Different Age Groups

12.1 Children and Adolescents

Promoting kidney health in children and adolescents begins with establishing healthy habits. Encourage them to drink plenty of water, limit sugary drinks, and maintain a balanced diet rich in fruits, vegetables, and whole grains. Emphasize the importance of regular physical activity to support overall health, including kidney function. Regular check-ups with a pediatrician can help monitor growth and identify any potential kidney-related issues early on.

12.2 Young Adults

As young adults navigate the transition to adulthood, they should prioritize kidney health by maintaining a healthy lifestyle. This includes staying well-hydrated, following a balanced diet low in sodium, and engaging in regular exercise. Young adults should be cautious about alcohol consumption and avoid smoking, as these habits can have long-term negative effects on kidney health. Regular check-ups with a healthcare provider can help assess kidney function and address any concerns.

12.3 Adults

Adults of all ages should maintain kidney health through healthy lifestyle choices. Follow a balanced diet that includes nutrient-rich foods and limits sodium, saturated fats, and added sugars. Stay physically active and manage stress effectively. It is crucial to monitor blood pressure, blood sugar levels, and cholesterol levels regularly, as these can impact kidney health. Avoid smoking and limit alcohol consumption. If taking any medications, follow healthcare provider's guidance and be aware of potential effects on kidney function.

12.4 Seniors

In the senior years, maintaining kidney health becomes even more important. Seniors should prioritize hydration, as aging can affect the body's ability to retain water. Be mindful of medication use and potential interactions with kidney function. Maintain a balanced diet that focuses on kidney-friendly foods and supports overall health. Regular check-ups, including kidney function tests, are essential for monitoring kidney health in seniors.

12.5 Pregnancy and Kidney Health

During pregnancy, kidney health is crucial for both the mother and the developing baby. Pregnant individuals should attend prenatal care visits regularly to monitor blood pressure and kidney function. Follow healthcare provider's guidance on nutrition, including prenatal vitamins, and maintain proper hydration. Any concerns or symptoms related to kidney health during pregnancy should be promptly discussed with a healthcare provider.

12.6 Chronic Conditions and Kidney Health

Individuals with chronic conditions such as diabetes, high blood pressure, or cardiovascular disease should take extra care to manage these conditions effectively. Follow healthcare provider's guidance on medications, lifestyle modifications, and regular check-ups to minimize the impact on kidney health. These individuals should work closely with healthcare providers to monitor kidney function and implement strategies to prevent or slow the progression of kidney disease.

Chapter 13: Common Myths and Misconceptions about Kidney Health

13.1 Myth: Drinking excessive amounts of water will cleanse the kidneys.

Fact: While staying properly hydrated is important for kidney health, drinking excessive amounts of water will not necessarily cleanse the kidneys more effectively. The kidneys naturally filter waste products from the blood, and drinking a moderate amount of water is sufficient to support their function. It is important to maintain a balance and drink an adequate amount of water throughout the day without overdoing it.

13.2 Myth: Consuming large amounts of protein is harmful to the kidneys.

Fact: While excessive protein intake can be taxing on the kidneys, moderate protein consumption is generally safe and important for overall health. It is important to maintain a balanced diet that includes an appropriate amount of protein. If you have existing kidney disease or compromised kidney function, it is recommended to consult with a healthcare professional or registered dietitian to determine the appropriate protein intake for your specific condition.

13.3 Myth: Kidney disease only affects older individuals.

Fact: While kidney disease is more prevalent in older individuals, it can affect people of all ages, including children and young adults. Various factors, including genetics, underlying health conditions, and lifestyle choices, can contribute to kidney disease at any age. It is important for individuals of all age groups to be aware of and prioritize kidney health.

13.4 Myth: Drinking herbal teas and supplements can reverse kidney disease.

Fact: While certain herbal teas and supplements may have health benefits, there is no cure for chronic kidney disease. It is important to approach any claims of reversing kidney disease with caution. Managing kidney disease typically involves a combination of medical treatments, lifestyle modifications, and adherence to a kidney-friendly diet. A healthcare professional should be consulted to determine the best management techniques.

13.5 Myth: Only people with high blood pressure or diabetes are at risk for kidney disease.

Fact: While high blood pressure and diabetes are common risk factors for kidney disease, there are other factors that can contribute to kidney damage. These include obesity, smoking, family history of kidney disease, certain medications, and certain medical conditions. It is important to be aware of these risk factors and take steps to mitigate them through healthy lifestyle choices and regular medical check-ups.

13.6 Myth: A kidney-friendly diet is too restrictive and lacking in flavor.

Fact: A kidney-friendly diet can be both nutritious and flavorful. While there may be some limitations on certain foods and nutrients, there are still plenty of delicious options available. The key is to focus on fresh fruits, vegetables, whole grains, lean proteins, and kidney-friendly herbs and spices. With creative cooking techniques and flavorful seasonings, you can enjoy a wide variety of tasty and kidney-friendly meals.

13.7 Myth: Kidney disease is always accompanied by noticeable symptoms.

Fact: In the early stages, kidney disease often does not present noticeable symptoms. It can progress silently, making regular check-ups and kidney function tests important for early detection. Symptoms may only become apparent in the later stages of kidney disease. Therefore, it is essential to monitor kidney health through routine medical evaluations, especially if you have risk factors or a family history of kidney disease.

Chapter 14: Additional Resources and Support for Kidney Health

14.1 Healthcare Providers and Specialists

Your primary care physician is an important resource for managing your overall health, including kidney health. They can provide routine check-ups, monitor your kidney function, and offer guidance on maintaining a healthy lifestyle. In some cases, they may refer you to a nephrologist, a physician specializing in kidney health, for further evaluation and treatment if needed. Nephrologists are well-versed in kidney diseases and can provide specialized care and recommendations.

14.2 Registered Dietitians

Registered dietitians can play a significant role in managing kidney health through diet and nutrition. They can help you develop a personalized meal plan that aligns with your specific kidney health needs, taking into consideration factors such as protein intake, sodium restriction, and potassium control. Registered dietitians can also provide education, support, and guidance on making kidney-friendly food choices.

14.3 Support Groups and Online Communities

Joining support groups and online communities can provide a sense of belonging, encouragement, and information sharing. Connecting with others who are experiencing similar challenges or have firsthand knowledge of kidney health can be empowering and comforting. These groups can offer a platform to ask questions, share experiences, and gain support from others who understand the journey.

14.4 Kidney Foundations and Organizations

Numerous kidney foundations and organizations are dedicated to promoting kidney health, raising awareness, and providing valuable resources. These organizations offer educational materials, research updates, and access to additional support services. Examples include the National Kidney Foundation, the American Association of Kidney Patients, and the Kidney Health Initiative. Exploring their websites or reaching out to them can provide valuable information and resources.

14.5 Educational Materials and Websites

Educational materials and reputable websites are excellent sources of information on kidney health. They can offer comprehensive information about kidney diseases, risk factors, preventive measures, and treatment options. Websites such as those of kidney foundations, healthcare institutions, and government health agencies often provide accurate and up-to-date information on kidney health.

14.6 Local Health Programs and Community Centers

Check with your local health programs and community centers for resources and events related to kidney health. They may offer educational sessions, workshops, or support groups that focus on kidney health. These programs can provide opportunities for learning, networking, and engaging with healthcare professionals and fellow individuals interested in maintaining kidney health.

14.7 National Kidney Month and Awareness Campaigns

National Kidney Month, observed in March, is an annual campaign dedicated to raising awareness about kidney health and diseases. During this month, various events, educational initiatives, and screenings are organized to promote kidney health. Stay informed about these campaigns and participate in activities to enhance your understanding and contribute to the broader kidney health community.

14.8 Books and Publications

There are numerous books and publications available that provide in-depth knowledge on kidney health, kidney diseases, and maintaining optimal kidney function. Look for reputable resources written by healthcare professionals, researchers, or individuals with expertise in kidney health. These resources can offer comprehensive information and insights to support your journey towards better kidney health.

Conclusion

Conclusion

A kidney-friendly diet plays a crucial role in maintaining optimal kidney health. Focus on consuming a balanced and nutritious diet that includes fresh fruits, vegetables, whole grains, lean proteins, and limited sodium, while also considering individual dietary restrictions and preferences.

Staying well-hydrated is essential for supporting kidney function. Aim to drink an adequate amount of water throughout the day, keeping in mind your individual needs and any specific recommendations from healthcare providers.

Regular physical activity, in conjunction with a healthy diet, can contribute to overall kidney health. Engage in moderate-intensity exercises such as walking, swimming, or cycling for at least 30 minutes most days of the week.

Manage and control conditions such as high blood pressure, diabetes, and obesity, as they can have a significant impact on kidney health. Regular check-ups, medication adherence, and lifestyle modifications are key in managing these conditions effectively.

Avoid smoking and limit alcohol consumption, as both habits can negatively affect kidney health and overall well-being.

Stay informed and seek reputable resources to debunk myths and misconceptions surrounding kidney health. Educating yourself empowers you to make informed decisions and take appropriate actions to maintain optimal kidney function.

Make use of the tools and systems of support that are at your disposal.. Healthcare providers, registered dietitians, support groups, and organizations dedicated to kidney health can provide valuable guidance, education, and assistance on your kidney health journey.

Remember, prioritizing kidney health is a lifelong commitment. Regular check-ups, screenings, and discussions with healthcare providers are essential for monitoring kidney function and addressing any concerns or changes. By implementing the knowledge and practices outlined in this book, you can take control of your kidney health and reduce the risk of kidney-related complications.

We hope this book has served as a comprehensive guide to understanding, maintaining, and promoting kidney health. By incorporating the recommendations, adopting a kidney-friendly lifestyle, and utilizing the available resources, you are taking significant steps toward preserving the well-being of your kidneys.

Here's to a future of vibrant kidney health and overall wellness. Stay committed, stay informed, and stay proactive on your journey to optimal kidney health.

Bonus

Meal Planning and Shopping Tips

Breakfast
- Oatmeal with fruit and nuts
- Yogurt with granola and berries
- Scrambled eggs with whole-wheat toast
- On whole-wheat bread, a peanut butter and banana sandwich is made.
- Whole-wheat waffles with fruit and syrup

Lunch
- Salad with grilled chicken or fish
- Soup and a sandwich
- Leftovers from dinner
- Tuna salad sandwich on whole-wheat bread
- Veggie wrap

Dinner
- Grilled salmon with roasted vegetables
- Chicken stir-fry with brown rice
- Lentil soup
- Turkey burgers on whole-wheat buns
- Vegetarian chili

Snacks
- Fruit
- Yogurt
- Nuts
- Hard-boiled eggs
- Trail mix

Shopping Tips
- Look for foods that are low in sodium, potassium, and phosphorus.
- Choose fresh fruits and vegetables over canned or frozen fruits and vegetables.
- Read food labels carefully to make sure you are choosing the right foods.

- Ask your doctor or a registered dietitian for more specific dietary recommendations.

Here are some additional tips for meal planning for seniors with renal disease:

- Make sure to eat regular meals and snacks throughout the day.
- Instead of salt, use herbs and spices to season your food.
- Use healthier fats when cooking, like canola or olive oil.
- Limit your intake of processed foods.
- Drink plenty of water.

Following these tips can help you create a healthy and delicious meal plan that is tailored to your individual needs.

Here is a sample shopping list for a week:

- Fruits: bananas, apples, oranges, grapes, berries
- Vegetables: broccoli, cauliflower, carrots, celery, spinach
- Protein: chicken, fish, tofu, beans, eggs
- Carbohydrates: whole-wheat bread, brown rice, pasta
- Dairy: low-fat milk, yogurt, cheese
- Other: nuts, seeds, oils, herbs, spices

Exercise and physical activity

1. Walking:A low-impact activity that is easy on the joints is walking. It can be done indoors or outdoors, and it can be as simple as walking around the block or taking a brisk walk in the park.

2. Water aerobics: Water aerobics is a great way to get exercise without putting stress on your joints. It is also a good way to cool off on hot days.

3. Tai chi: Tai chi is a gentle form of exercise that combines slow, flowing movements with meditation. It is a fantastic way to increase flexibility and balance.

4. Yoga: Yoga is another gentle form of exercise that can improve balance, flexibility, and strength. You can find the right kind of yoga for you because there are numerous variations.

5. Strength training: Strength training exercises can help to build muscle and improve bone health. These exercises can be done with weights, resistance bands, or your own body weight.

6. Cycling: Cycling is a great way to get exercise and enjoy the outdoors. It is a low-impact exercise that is easy on the joints.

7. Dancing: Dancing is a fun and social way to get exercise. There are many different types of dancing, so you can find one that you enjoy.

8. Hiking: Hiking is a great way to get exercise and enjoy the outdoors. It is a moderate-impact exercise that can be challenging but rewarding.

9. Swimming: Swimming is a great way to get exercise and cool off on hot days. It is a low-impact exercise that is easy on the joints.

10. Martial arts: Martial arts can help to improve balance, coordination, and strength. They can also be a great way to learn self-defense.

These are just a few examples of physical activities and exercises that are good for seniors with renal disease. Before beginning any new exercise program, it's important to consult your doctor. They can help you to choose the right activities for your individual needs and fitness level.

Here are some additional tips for exercising with renal disease:

- Start out slowly, then gradually increase the length and intensity of your workouts.

- When taking breaks, pay attention to what your body needs.
- Keep hydrated by consuming lots of liquids.
- Wear comfortable clothing and shoes.
- Choose activities that you enjoy and that are safe for your individual needs.

With a little planning and effort, you can find physical activities that are enjoyable and beneficial for your health.

www.ingramcontent.com/pod-product-compliance
Lightning Source LLC
Chambersburg PA
CBHW062240290526
45794CB00006B/2352